DASH DIET COOKBOOK FOR ALZHEIMER'S

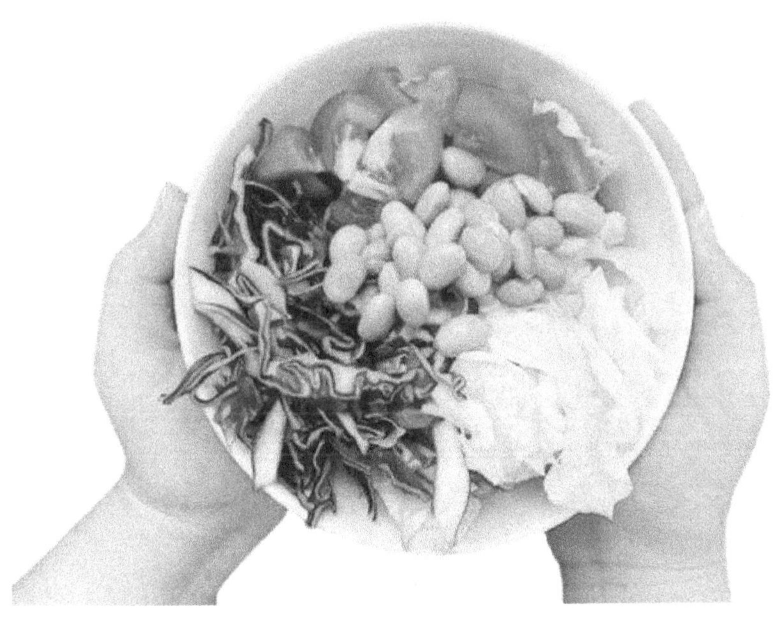

DR. VICKIE STOCK

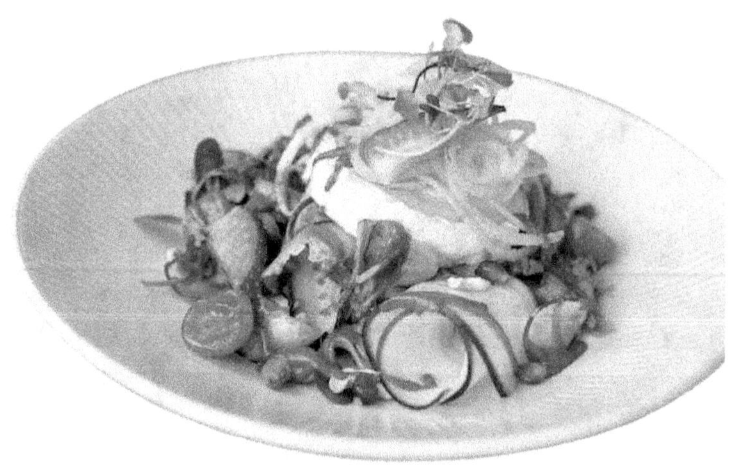

TABLE OF CONTENT

HOW TO USE THIS COOKBOOK

Introduction:

Begin by reading the cookbook's introduction to grasp its purpose and the DASH diet's tailored approach for Alzheimer's prevention.

Understand DASH Diet Principles:

Familiarize yourself with the core principles of the DASH diet, emphasizing whole foods like fruits, vegetables, lean proteins, and whole grains.

Navigate Recipe Sections:

Explore various recipe sections, including breakfast, lunch, dinner, snacks, desserts, and smoothies, tailoring your choices to specific times or preferences.

Review Recipe Headings:

Quickly identify suitable meals by reading recipe headings, helping you pinpoint recipes for specific meals or occasions.

Examine Nutritional Information: Prioritize recipes by checking nutritional information for calories, macronutrients, and essential vitamins, ensuring alignment with dietary goals.

Check Ingredient Accessibility:

Verify that listed ingredients are readily available. Modify or substitute based on preferences or dietary restrictions, ensuring a practical approach.

Follow Detailed Instructions:

Execute recipes step by step, adhering to cooking techniques, temperatures, and suggested times for optimal results.

Experiment with Flavor Profiles:

Enhance your culinary experience by experimenting with herbs, spices, and seasonings. Tailor flavors to suit personal taste preferences while staying within DASH diet guidelines.

Optimize Meal Planning:

Maximize the cookbook for effective meal planning, creating diverse daily or weekly plans by combining recipes for a well-rounded and nutritious diet.

- Monitor Cognitive Health:

Observe and track the impact of DASH diet recipes on cognitive health. Document any positive changes and, for personalized guidance, consult healthcare professionals.

CHAPTER ONE: Introduction

Overview of the DASH Diet for Alzheimer's Prevention

The DASH (Dietary Approaches to Stop Hypertension) Diet has gained widespread recognition for its cardiovascular benefits, but its impact on brain health, specifically in Alzheimer's prevention, is equally noteworthy. The core principles of the DASH Diet focus on promoting overall well-being, emphasizing nutrient-rich foods and limiting sodium intake.

Balanced Nutrition:

At the heart of the DASH Diet is a commitment to balanced and nutritious eating. It encourages the consumption of fruits, vegetables, lean proteins, whole grains, and low-fat dairy products. These elements provide essential vitamins, minerals, antioxidants, and fiber crucial for maintaining optimal cognitive function.

Blood Pressure Regulation:

One of the primary goals of the DASH Diet is to regulate blood pressure. By incorporating potassium-rich foods and reducing sodium intake, the diet helps maintain healthy blood vessels and improve blood flow. This vascular support is integral to preventing conditions that could contribute to cognitive decline, including Alzheimer's disease.

Inflammation Reduction:

Chronic inflammation is a known factor linked to various health issues, including cognitive decline. The DASH Diet, with its emphasis on anti-inflammatory foods like fruits, vegetables, and omega-3 fatty acids, aids in reducing inflammation throughout the body, promoting long-term brain health.

Stress on Heart-Healthy Fats:

The inclusion of heart-healthy fats, such as those found in nuts, seeds, and olive oil, is another distinctive feature of the DASH Diet. These fats contribute to overall cardiovascular health and, by extension, support brain function.

Impact on Cognitive Function:

Research suggests that adherence to the DASH Diet may be associated with a lower risk of cognitive decline and neurodegenerative diseases. The combination of nutrient-dense foods, blood pressure regulation, and anti-inflammatory properties creates a dietary foundation that may contribute to a healthier brain as individuals age.

The DASH Diet's comprehensive approach to nutrition, blood pressure regulation, and anti-inflammatory effects positions it as a valuable tool in the prevention of Alzheimer's disease and the maintenance of cognitive well-being.

Adopting the DASH Diet principles offers not only cardiovascular benefits but also a promising avenue for enhancing brain health.

Importance of Nutrition in Cognitive Health

The importance of nutrition in cognitive health cannot be overstated, as the food we consume plays a pivotal role in shaping the functionality and resilience of the brain. A well-balanced and nutrient-rich diet not only fuels our bodies but also provides the essential elements necessary for optimal cognitive function.

Nutrient Influence on Brain Structure:

The brain is a highly metabolically active organ, and its structure is influenced by the nutrients we consume. Essential vitamins, minerals, and omega-3 fatty acids contribute to the formation of neural pathways, the synthesis of neurotransmitters, and the overall maintenance of brain cells. Adequate nutrition is fundamental for sustaining the structural integrity of the brain.

Energy Supply for Cognitive Processes:

The brain requires a substantial amount of energy to carry out its complex cognitive processes. Glucose, derived from carbohydrates, serves as the primary energy source for the brain. A diet rich in complex carbohydrates ensures a steady supply of glucose, supporting concentration, memory, and overall cognitive performance.

Antioxidants and Neuroprotection:

Antioxidant-rich foods, including fruits and vegetables, play a crucial role in protecting the brain from oxidative stress. The brain is particularly vulnerable to oxidative damage due to its high oxygen consumption. Antioxidants neutralize free radicals, preventing potential harm to brain cells and supporting long-term cognitive health.

Inflammation Management:

Chronic inflammation has been linked to cognitive decline and neurodegenerative diseases. Nutrition plays a vital role in either promoting or mitigating inflammation. Diets rich in anti-inflammatory foods, such as fatty fish, nuts, and leafy greens, contribute to a healthier inflammatory response, reducing the risk of cognitive impairment.

Impact of Micronutrients on Mental Health:

Micronutrients like B vitamins, zinc, and magnesium are essential for mental well-being. They contribute to the regulation of mood, sleep, and stress response. Inadequate levels of these micronutrients can adversely affect mental health and potentially contribute to cognitive disorders.

CHAPTER TWO: Dash Diet Essentials

Core Principles and Guidelines

The core principles and guidelines of the DASH (Dietary Approaches to Stop Hypertension) Diet are rooted in promoting cardiovascular health, but their impact extends to various facets of overall well-being, including cognitive health.

These principles emphasize a balanced and nutrient-rich approach to eating, aiming to lower blood pressure, reduce the risk of chronic diseases, and contribute to optimal brain function.

1. Emphasis on Fruits and Vegetables:

A cornerstone of the DASH Diet is the promotion of a high intake of fruits and vegetables. These foods provide essential vitamins, minerals, antioxidants, and fiber crucial for maintaining overall health. In the context of cognitive well-being, the nutrient density of fruits and vegetables contributes to the nourishment of brain cells and the prevention of oxidative stress.

2. Inclusion of Lean Proteins:

The DASH Diet encourages the consumption of lean proteins such as poultry, fish, beans, and nuts. Proteins are essential for the synthesis of neurotransmitters and the repair and maintenance of brain cells. The inclusion of lean proteins supports cognitive functions such as memory and concentration.

3. Whole Grains for Sustained Energy:

Whole grains, another fundamental component of the DASH Diet, provide a steady supply of complex carbohydrates, ensuring a sustained release of glucose into the bloodstream. This helps maintain consistent energy levels for the brain, supporting cognitive processes throughout the day.

4. Moderate Dairy Intake:

The diet recommends moderate consumption of low-fat dairy products, contributing to the intake of calcium and vitamin D. These nutrients are essential for maintaining bone health, and emerging research suggests potential connections between bone health and cognitive function.

5. Sodium Moderation:

To address hypertension, the DASH Diet advocates for the moderation of sodium intake. By reducing sodium levels, the diet helps maintain healthy blood vessels, promoting optimal blood flow to the brain and reducing the risk of cognitive decline.

6. Healthy Fats in Moderation:

While the DASH Diet emphasizes healthy fats like those found in nuts, seeds, and olive oil, it suggests moderation to maintain overall caloric balance. These fats contribute to cardiovascular health, indirectly supporting cognitive function.

Benefits of the DASH Diet for Brain Health

The DASH (Dietary Approaches to Stop Hypertension) Diet, renowned for its cardiovascular benefits, also presents a wealth of advantages for brain health. The diet's emphasis on nutrient-dense foods and specific dietary patterns contributes to cognitive well-being, potentially lowering the risk of neurodegenerative diseases and supporting optimal brain function.

1. Nutrient-Rich Foods for Cognitive Nourishment:

A primary benefit of the DASH Diet for brain health lies in its promotion of nutrient-rich foods. Fruits, vegetables, whole grains, and lean proteins provide a spectrum of vitamins, minerals, antioxidants, and essential fatty acids crucial for the nourishment and protection of brain cells.

2. Blood Pressure Regulation and Cognitive Protection:

The DASH Diet's effectiveness in regulating blood pressure has direct implications for brain health. By supporting healthy blood vessels and improving blood flow, the diet contributes to the prevention of conditions that may lead to cognitive decline, including Alzheimer's disease.

3. Reduction of Oxidative Stress:

Oxidative stress, resulting from an imbalance between free radicals and antioxidants in the body, is a contributor to age-related cognitive decline. The DASH Diet's emphasis on antioxidant-rich foods, such as berries and leafy greens, helps counteract oxidative stress, providing neuroprotective benefits.

4. Anti-Inflammatory Effects:

Chronic inflammation is increasingly recognized as a factor in cognitive decline and neurodegenerative diseases. The DASH Diet's focus on anti-inflammatory foods, including fatty fish and nuts, contributes to reducing inflammation in the body, potentially safeguarding the brain from harmful effects.

5. Balanced Macronutrient Intake:

The DASH Diet encourages a balanced intake of macronutrients, ensuring an adequate supply of carbohydrates, proteins, and healthy fats. This balance supports energy metabolism and neurotransmitter synthesis, contributing to overall cognitive function.

6. Maintenance of Vascular Health:

Healthy blood vessels are vital for proper brain function. The DASH Diet's impact on vascular health, driven by reduced sodium intake and increased potassium consumption, plays a crucial role in preserving optimal blood circulation to the brain.

CHAPTER THREE: Cooking Tips and Guidelines for Brain-Healthy Meals

Creating brain-healthy meals involves more than just assembling ingredients. It's about choosing nutrient-dense foods and employing cooking methods that preserve and enhance their cognitive benefits. The following tips and guidelines, coupled with effective meal planning strategies, can contribute to a brain-boosting culinary experience.

1. Prioritize Nutrient-Dense Ingredients

Colorful Variety: Opt for a diverse range of colorful fruits and vegetables to ensure a spectrum of essential nutrients and antioxidants.

Omega-3 Rich Foods: Incorporate fatty fish, flaxseeds, and walnuts to provide omega-3 fatty acids vital for brain health.

Whole Grains: Choose whole grains like quinoa, brown rice, and oats to supply a steady release of energy and support cognitive function.

2. Mindful Cooking Techniques

Steam and Saute: Use gentle cooking methods like steaming and sautéing to preserve the nutritional value of vegetables and prevent nutrient loss.

Limit Processed Foods: Minimize the use of processed ingredients high in additives and preservatives, as they may contribute to cognitive decline.

Herbs and Spices: Enhance flavor with herbs and spices, known for their antioxidant and anti-inflammatory properties. Examples include turmeric, rosemary, and cinnamon.

3. Healthy Fats and Protein Balance

Good Fats: Include sources of healthy fats such as avocados, olive oil, and nuts to support brain function.

Lean Proteins: Prioritize lean protein sources like poultry, fish, beans, and legumes for sustained energy without excessive saturated fats.

Plant-Based Options: Explore plant-based protein alternatives like tofu and legumes, offering diverse nutrients without compromising brain health.

4. Hydration Matters

Water Intake: Stay adequately hydrated, as dehydration can impair cognitive function. Include herbal teas, infused water, and hydrating fruits like watermelon.

1. Balanced Meals Throughout the Day

Breakfast Boost: Start the day with a nutrient-packed breakfast, incorporating fruits, whole grains, and a source of protein.

Protein at Every Meal: Include a source of protein in every meal to support muscle and brain health.

Midday Energy Snacks: Opt for nutrient-rich snacks, such as nuts, seeds, or yogurt, to maintain steady energy levels between meals.

2. Weekly Meal Prep

Batch Cooking: Plan and prepare ingredients in batches for the week to streamline the cooking process and ensure convenient access to brain-healthy options.

Diverse Recipes: Rotate through a variety of brain-boosting recipes to keep meals interesting and nutritionally rich.

3. Mindful Portions

Balanced Portions: Pay attention to portion sizes, ensuring a balance of macronutrients without excessive caloric intake.

Colorful Plate: Aim for a colorful plate with a mix of vegetables, lean proteins, and whole grains to maximize nutritional diversity.

4. Adapt to Personal Preferences and Dietary Needs

Flexibility: Tailor meal plans to individual preferences, accommodating dietary restrictions and preferences to ensure a sustainable and enjoyable approach to brain-healthy eating.

By incorporating these cooking tips and meal plan strategies, you embark on a journey to not only enhance brain health but also cultivate a sustainable and enjoyable approach to nourishing your body and mind. The key lies in the mindful selection of ingredients, thoughtful cooking techniques, and a well-structured meal plan that aligns with your individual needs and goals.

CHAPTER FOUR: Brain-Boosting Ingredients: Harnessing the Power of Antioxidants

Understanding the impact of nutrition on cognitive health opens the door to a world of brain-boosting ingredients. Antioxidants, in particular, play a crucial role in supporting brain function and protecting against oxidative stress. Let's delve into the rich array of brain-boosting ingredients and unravel the roles of antioxidants in promoting cognitive well-being.

1. Berries: Nature's Antioxidant Powerhouses

- Blueberries: Packed with anthocyanins, blueberries are potent antioxidants that may improve memory and cognitive function by enhancing signaling in the brain.

- Strawberries: Rich in vitamin C and manganese, strawberries contribute to a healthy brain by reducing oxidative stress.

2. Fatty Fish: Omega-3 Fatty Acids for Cognitive Vitality

- Salmon: Abundant in omega-3 fatty acids, especially DHA, salmon supports brain structure and function, promoting optimal cognitive performance.

- Walnuts: These nuts are a plant-based source of omega-3 fatty acids, aiding in improved memory and cognitive function.

3. Dark Leafy Greens: Nutrient-Rich Brain Allies

- Kale: Loaded with antioxidants, kale supports brain health by providing essential nutrients like vitamin K, A, and C.
- Spinach: High in folate and iron, spinach supports cognitive development and may reduce the risk of age-related cognitive decline.

4. Avocados: Healthy Fats and Antioxidants

- Monounsaturated Fats: Avocados contain monounsaturated fats that support healthy blood flow, vital for maintaining optimal brain function.
- Vitamin E: A potent antioxidant in avocados, vitamin E protects cells from oxidative stress.

5. Nuts and Seeds: Brain-Friendly Nutrients

- Almonds: Rich in vitamin E, almonds provide antioxidant protection and may contribute to cognitive function as part of a balanced diet.
- Chia Seeds: Packed with omega-3 fatty acids, fiber, and antioxidants, chia seeds support overall brain health.

6. Turmeric: Curcumin's Neuroprotective Role

Curcumin: The active compound in turmeric, curcumin, has anti-inflammatory and antioxidant benefits, potentially promoting neuroplasticity.

7. Broccoli: Brain-Nourishing Nutrients

Vitamin K: Broccoli is a rich source of vitamin K, important for forming sphingolipids, a type of fat densely packed into brain cells.

Antioxidants: Broccoli contains various antioxidants, including vitamin C, beta-carotene, and sulforaphane, which may have protective effects.

8. Dark Chocolate: Indulgence with Cognitive Perks

Flavanols: Dark chocolate is rich in flavanols, antioxidants that may improve blood flow to the brain and enhance cognitive function.

9. Coffee: A Stimulating Antioxidant Source

Caffeine: Coffee, in moderation, contains caffeine, which can improve mood, reaction time, and general mental function.

Chlorogenic Acids: These antioxidants in coffee may have neuroprotective effects.

10. Green Tea: L-Theanine and Antioxidant Synergy

L-Theanine: Green tea contains L-theanine, an amino acid that, when combined with caffeine, can have positive effects on cognitive performance.

Catechins: Green tea is rich in catechins, powerful antioxidants that may provide neuroprotective benefits.

The Role of Antioxidants in Brain Health

Neutralizing Free Radicals: Antioxidants combat free radicals, unstable molecules that can cause cellular damage, including in the brain.

Reducing Inflammation: Many antioxidants have anti-inflammatory properties, potentially protecting the brain from chronic inflammation.

Supporting Neuroplasticity: Antioxidants may support neuroplasticity, the brain's ability to reorganize and form new connections.

Incorporating a diverse array of brain-boosting ingredients rich in antioxidants into your diet can contribute to cognitive well-being. These foods not only provide essential nutrients but also offer powerful protection against oxidative stress, supporting a healthy and resilient brain.

CHAPTER FIVE: Dash Diet Recipes for Alzheimer's

Breakfast Delight

1. Berry and Walnut Parfait

Ingredients:

- 1 cup non-fat Greek yogurt
- 1/2 cup mixed berries (blueberries, strawberries, raspberries)
- 2 tablespoons chopped walnuts
- 1 tablespoon honey
- 1/4 teaspoon vanilla extract

Instructions:

- In a serving glass, layer half of the Greek yogurt.
- Add half of the mixed berries on top.
- Sprinkle half of the chopped walnuts.
- Drizzle with half of the honey and a splash of vanilla extract.
- Repeat the layering process with the remaining ingredients.
- Serve immediately and enjoy this antioxidant-rich, protein-packed breakfast.

Nutritional Value:

- Calories: 300

- Protein: 20g

- Fiber: 5g

- Healthy Fats: 12g

Health Benefits:

- High in antioxidants from berries.

- Omega-3 fatty acids from walnuts support brain health.

- Greek yogurt provides probiotics for gut health.

Preparation Time: 5 minutes

2. Veggie and Feta Omelette

Ingredients:

- 2 large eggs

- 1/4 cup diced bell peppers (mixed colors)

- 1/4 cup diced tomatoes

- 2 tablespoons crumbled feta cheese

- 1 tablespoon chopped fresh basil

- Salt and pepper to taste

Instructions:

- Whisk eggs in a bowl and season with salt and pepper.

- Heat a non-stick skillet over medium heat.

- Pour the whisked eggs into the skillet.

- Sprinkle bell peppers, tomatoes, feta cheese, and fresh basil evenly over one half of the omelette.

- Once the edges are set, fold the other half over the filling.

- Cook for an additional minute until the cheese is melted.

- Slide onto a plate, slice, and serve.

Nutritional Value:

- Calories: 250

- Protein: 18g

- Fiber: 3g

- Calcium: 150mg

Health Benefits:

- Bell peppers provide vitamin C.

- Tomatoes offer lycopene, beneficial for brain health.

- Feta cheese adds a dose of calcium.

Preparation Time: 10 minutes

3. Overnight Chia Seed Pudding

Ingredients:

- 2 tablespoons chia seeds

- 1/2 cup unsweetened almond milk

- 1/4 teaspoon vanilla extract

- 1 tablespoon maple syrup

- Sliced almonds and fresh berries for topping

Instructions:

- In a jar, mix chia seeds, almond milk, vanilla extract, and maple syrup.
- Stir well, ensuring the chia seeds are fully immersed in the liquid.
- Seal the jar and refrigerate overnight or for at least 4 hours.
- Before serving, stir the pudding to avoid clumps.
- Top with sliced almonds and fresh berries.

Nutritional Value:

- Calories: 200
- Protein: 6g
- Fiber: 10g
- Omega-3 Fatty Acids: 2.5g

Health Benefits:

- Chia seeds are rich in omega-3 fatty acids.
- Almond milk provides vitamin E.
- Berries add antioxidants for brain health.

Preparation Time: 5 minutes (plus overnight chilling)

4. Spinach and Feta Breakfast Wrap

Ingredients:

- 1 whole-grain tortilla
- 2 large eggs, scrambled
- 1 cup fresh spinach leaves
- 2 tablespoons crumbled feta cheese
- 1/4 cup diced tomatoes
- Salt and pepper to taste

Instructions:

- Heat the tortilla in a dry skillet or microwave until warm.
- In the same skillet, sauté spinach until wilted.
- Spread the scrambled eggs over the tortilla.
- Layer with sautéed spinach, feta cheese, and diced tomatoes.
- Season with salt and pepper.
- Fold the sides of the tortilla and roll it up into a wrap.
- Slice in half and serve.

Nutritional Value:

- Calories: 300
- Protein: 18g
- Fiber: 5g
- Iron: 3mg

Health Benefits:

- Spinach provides iron for improved cognitive function.
- Feta cheese contributes calcium.

Preparation Time: 15 minutes

5. Quinoa Breakfast Bowl

Ingredients:

- 1/2 cup cooked quinoa
- 1/4 cup unsweetened Greek yogurt
- 1 tablespoon almond butter
- 1/2 banana, sliced
- 1 tablespoon chia seeds
- Drizzle of honey

Instructions:

- In a bowl, layer cooked quinoa.
- Top with Greek yogurt and almond butter.
- Add sliced banana and sprinkle chia seeds.
- Drizzle with honey for sweetness.
- Mix before eating to combine flavors.

Nutritional Value:

- Calories: 350

- Protein: 15g

- Fiber: 7g

- Potassium: 450mg

Health Benefits:

- Quinoa provides a complete protein source.

- Almond butter adds healthy fats.

- Banana contributes potassium.

Preparation Time: 10 minutes

6. Blueberry Oatmeal Muffins

Ingredients:

- 1 cup rolled oats

- 1/2 cup whole wheat flour

- 1/2 cup almond flour

- 1 teaspoon baking powder

- 1/2 teaspoon cinnamon

- 1/4 teaspoon salt

- 2 ripe bananas, mashed

- 2 large eggs

- 1/4 cup honey

- 1/4 cup Greek yogurt

- 1 cup fresh blueberries

Instructions:

- Preheat the oven to 350°F (175°C) and line a muffin tin with paper liners.
- In a bowl, mix oats, whole wheat flour, almond flour, baking powder, cinnamon, and salt.
- In another bowl, whisk mashed bananas, eggs, honey, and Greek yogurt.
- Combine wet and dry ingredients, then fold in blueberries.
- Spoon the batter into muffin cups, filling each about two-thirds full.
- Bake for 18-20 minutes or until a toothpick comes out clean.
- Allow to cool before serving.

Nutritional Value:

- Calories: 180 (per muffin)
- Protein: 5g
- Fiber: 4g
- Antioxidants from blueberries

Health Benefits:

- Oats provide soluble fiber for heart and brain health.
- Blueberries offer antioxidants for cognitive support.

Preparation Time: 25 minutes

7. Sweet Potato and Kale Breakfast Hash

Ingredients:

- 1 medium sweet potato, diced
- 1 cup kale, finely chopped
- 1/2 onion, diced
- 2 cloves garlic, minced
- 2 eggs
- 1 tablespoon olive oil
- Salt and pepper to taste

Instructions:

- Heat olive oil in a skillet over medium heat.
- Add diced sweet potatoes and cook until they begin to soften.
- Add diced onions and minced garlic, sauté until fragrant.
- Stir in chopped kale and continue cooking until kale is wilted.
- Make two wells in the hash and crack an egg into each.
- Cover the skillet and cook until the eggs are cooked to your liking.
- Season with salt and pepper, and serve warm.

Nutritional Value:

- Calories: 320

- Protein: 13g

- Fiber: 6g

- Vitamin A: 200% DV

Health Benefits:

- Sweet potatoes offer vitamin A for eye health.

- Kale provides antioxidants and essential nutrients.

Preparation Time: 20 minutes

8. Avocado and Smoked Salmon Toast

Ingredients:

- 2 slices whole-grain bread

- 1 ripe avocado

- 4 ounces smoked salmon

- 1 tablespoon lemon juice

- 1 tablespoon fresh dill, chopped

- Salt and pepper to taste

Instructions:

- Toast the whole-grain bread slices.

- Mash the ripe avocado and spread it evenly on the toasted bread.

- Lay smoked salmon slices on top of the mashed avocado.

- Drizzle lemon juice over the salmon.

- Sprinkle chopped fresh dill, salt, and pepper.

- Serve as an open-faced sandwich.

Nutritional Value:

- Calories: 340

- Protein: 20g

- Healthy Fats: 15g

- Omega-3 Fatty Acids: 1.5g

Health Benefits:

- Avocado provides healthy monounsaturated fats.

- Smoked salmon offers omega-3 fatty acids for brain health.

Preparation Time: 10 minutes

9. Almond and Berry Smoothie Bowl

Ingredients:

- 1 cup unsweetened almond milk

- 1/2 cup frozen mixed berries (blueberries, strawberries, raspberries)

- 1 ripe banana, frozen

- 2 tablespoons almond butter

- 1 tablespoon chia seeds

- Fresh berries and sliced almonds for topping

Instructions:

- In a blender, combine almond milk, frozen berries, frozen banana, almond butter, and chia seeds.
- Blend until smooth and creamy.
- Pour the smoothie into a bowl.
- Top with fresh berries and sliced almonds for added texture and nutrients.
- Enjoy this nutrient-packed, brain-boosting smoothie bowl.

Nutritional Value:

- Calories: 320
- Protein: 8g
- Fiber: 10g
- Vitamin E: 5mg

Health Benefits:

- Almond butter provides vitamin E, an antioxidant.
- Chia seeds contribute omega-3 fatty acids.
- Berries offer a mix of antioxidants.

Preparation Time: 5 minutes

10. Mediterranean Egg Muffins

Ingredients:

- 4 large eggs
- 1/2 cup cherry tomatoes, halved
- 1/4 cup feta cheese, crumbled
- 2 tablespoons Kalamata olives, chopped
- 1 tablespoon fresh oregano, chopped
- Salt and pepper to taste

Instructions:

- Preheat the oven to 350°F (175°C) and grease a muffin tin.
- In a bowl, whisk the eggs and season with salt and pepper.
- Divide the whisked eggs evenly among the muffin cups.
- Top each with cherry tomatoes, feta cheese, Kalamata olives, and fresh oregano.
- Bake for 15-18 minutes or until the egg is set.
- Allow to cool slightly before removing from the muffin tin.
- Serve these Mediterranean-inspired egg muffins warm.

Nutritional Value:

- Calories: 180 (per muffin)
- Protein: 10g
- Healthy Fats: 12g

- Vitamin C: 12mg

Health Benefits:

- Tomatoes provide vitamin C and lycopene.
- Feta cheese adds calcium.
- Olives contribute healthy monounsaturated fats.

Preparation Time: 20 minutes

Lunchtime Wellness

11. Grilled Salmon Salad

Ingredients:

- 6 ounces salmon fillet
- 2 cups mixed salad greens
- 1 cup cherry tomatoes, halved
- 1/2 cucumber, sliced
- 1/4 cup red onion, thinly sliced
- 1 tablespoon olive oil
- 1 tablespoon balsamic vinegar
- Salt and pepper to taste
- Fresh lemon wedges for serving

Instructions:

- Preheat the grill or grill pan over medium-high heat.

- Season the salmon fillet with salt and pepper.

- Grill the salmon for 3-4 minutes per side or until cooked to your liking.

- In a large bowl, toss the salad greens, cherry tomatoes, cucumber, and red onion.

- Drizzle with olive oil and balsamic vinegar, tossing to coat.

- Place the grilled salmon on top of the salad.

- Serve with fresh lemon wedges for extra flavor.

Nutritional Value:

- Calories: 400

- Protein: 30g

- Omega-3 Fatty Acids: 2.5g

- Vitamin C: 30mg

Health Benefits:

- Salmon provides omega-3 fatty acids for brain health.

- Salad greens offer a mix of vitamins and antioxidants.

Preparation Time: 20 minutes

12. Quinoa and Vegetable Stir-Fry

Ingredients:

- 1 cup quinoa, cooked

- 1 cup broccoli florets

- 1 bell pepper, thinly sliced (any color)
- 1 carrot, julienned
- 1/2 cup snap peas, trimmed
- 2 cloves garlic, minced
- 2 tablespoons low-sodium soy sauce
- 1 tablespoon sesame oil
- 1 teaspoon fresh ginger, grated
- 1 tablespoon sesame seeds for garnish

Instructions:

- In a large skillet or wok, heat sesame oil over medium-high heat.
- Add minced garlic and grated ginger, stir-frying for 30 seconds.
- Add broccoli, bell pepper, carrot, and snap peas to the skillet.
- Stir-fry for 5-7 minutes until vegetables are tender-crisp.
- Add cooked quinoa to the skillet, tossing to combine.
- Pour in low-sodium soy sauce, continuing to stir-fry for an additional 2-3 minutes.
- Garnish with sesame seeds before serving.

Nutritional Value:

- Calories: 350
- Protein: 12g

- Fiber: 7g

- Iron: 3mg

Health Benefits:

- Quinoa provides a complete protein source.

- Vegetables offer a variety of vitamins and minerals.

Preparation Time: 25 minutes

13. Turkey and Avocado Wrap

Ingredients:

- 4 ounces lean turkey breast slices

- 1 whole-grain wrap

- 1/2 avocado, sliced

- 1/2 cup spinach leaves

- 1/4 cup shredded carrots

- 1 tablespoon hummus

- 1 teaspoon Dijon mustard

Instructions:

- Lay the whole-grain wrap flat on a clean surface.

- Spread hummus evenly over the wrap, leaving a border around the edges.

- Layer turkey slices, avocado slices, spinach leaves, and shredded carrots.

- Drizzle Dijon mustard over the ingredients.
- Roll the wrap tightly and slice it in half.
- Serve as a nutritious and satisfying lunch option.

Nutritional Value:

- Calories: 380
- Protein: 25g
- Fiber: 8g
- Healthy Fats: 15g

Health Benefits:

- Turkey provides lean protein.
- Avocado contributes healthy monounsaturated fats.
- Whole-grain wrap adds dietary fiber.

Preparation Time: 10 minutes

14. Lentil and Vegetable Soup

Ingredients:

- 1 cup dry green or brown lentils, rinsed
- 1 onion, chopped
- 2 carrots, diced
- 2 celery stalks, sliced
- 2 cloves garlic, minced
- 1 can (14 oz) diced tomatoes, undrained

- 6 cups low-sodium vegetable broth

- 1 teaspoon ground cumin

- 1/2 teaspoon smoked paprika

- Salt and pepper to taste

- Fresh parsley for garnish

Instructions:

- In a large pot, combine lentils, onion, carrots, celery, garlic, diced tomatoes, vegetable broth, cumin, and smoked paprika.

- Bring to a boil, then reduce heat and simmer for 25-30 minutes or until lentils are tender.

- Season with salt and pepper to taste.

- Ladle the soup into bowls and garnish with fresh parsley.

- Enjoy this hearty and nutrient-packed lentil soup.

Nutritional Value:

- Calories: 300

- Protein: 18g

- Fiber: 16g

- Iron: 4mg

Health Benefits:

- Lentils are rich in fiber and protein.

- Vegetables provide essential vitamins and minerals.
- The soup is low in saturated fat and high in dietary fiber.

Preparation Time: 40 minutes

15. Chickpea and Spinach Salad

Ingredients:

- 1 can (15 oz) chickpeas, drained and rinsed
- 2 cups fresh spinach leaves
- 1 cup cherry tomatoes, halved
- 1/2 cucumber, diced
- 1/4 cup red onion, finely chopped
- 2 tablespoons feta cheese, crumbled
- 1 tablespoon extra virgin olive oil
- 1 tablespoon balsamic vinegar
- 1 teaspoon Dijon mustard
- Salt and pepper to taste

Instructions:

- In a large bowl, combine chickpeas, spinach, cherry tomatoes, cucumber, red onion, and feta cheese.
- In a small bowl, whisk together olive oil, balsamic vinegar, Dijon mustard, salt, and pepper.
- Drizzle the dressing over the salad and toss to combine.

- Serve immediately as a refreshing and nutrient-packed salad.

Nutritional Value:

- Calories: 340
- Protein: 12g
- Fiber: 10g
- Healthy Fats: 10g

Health Benefits:

- Chickpeas provide plant-based protein and fiber.
- Spinach offers iron and other essential nutrients.
- Feta cheese adds calcium for bone health.

Preparation Time: 15 minutes

16. Quinoa Stuffed Bell Peppers

Ingredients:

- 4 bell peppers, halved and seeds removed
- 1 cup quinoa, cooked
- 1 can (15 oz) black beans, drained and rinsed
- 1 cup corn kernels (fresh or frozen)
- 1 cup diced tomatoes
- 1/2 cup diced red onion
- 1 teaspoon ground cumin
- 1/2 teaspoon chili powder

- Salt and pepper to taste
- Fresh cilantro for garnish

Instructions:

- Preheat the oven to 375°F (190°C).
- In a large bowl, combine cooked quinoa, black beans, corn, tomatoes, red onion, cumin, chili powder, salt, and pepper.
- Spoon the quinoa mixture into each bell pepper half.
- Place stuffed peppers in a baking dish.
- Cover with foil and bake for 25-30 minutes or until peppers are tender.
- Garnish with fresh cilantro before serving.

Nutritional Value:

- Calories: 320
- Protein: 14g
- Fiber: 9g
- Vitamin C: 120mg

Health Benefits:

- Quinoa offers a complete protein source.
- Bell peppers provide vitamin C and antioxidants.
- Black beans contribute fiber for digestive health.

Preparation Time: 40 minutes

17. Mediterranean Chickpea Bowl

Ingredients:

- 1 cup cooked quinoa
- 1 can (15 oz) chickpeas, drained and rinsed
- 1 cup cherry tomatoes, halved
- 1/2 cucumber, diced
- 1/4 cup Kalamata olives, sliced
- 2 tablespoons feta cheese, crumbled
- 1 tablespoon extra virgin olive oil
- 1 tablespoon lemon juice
- 1 teaspoon dried oregano
- Salt and pepper to taste

Instructions:

- In a bowl, combine cooked quinoa, chickpeas, cherry tomatoes, cucumber, Kalamata olives, and feta cheese.
- In a small bowl, whisk together olive oil, lemon juice, dried oregano, salt, and pepper.
- Drizzle the dressing over the bowl and toss gently to combine.
- Serve as a flavorful and satisfying Mediterranean-inspired lunch.

Nutritional Value:

- Calories: 380
- Protein: 14g
- Fiber: 9g
- Healthy Fats: 12g

Health Benefits:

- Chickpeas provide plant-based protein and fiber.
- Olive oil contributes heart-healthy monounsaturated fats.
- Mediterranean ingredients offer antioxidants.

Preparation Time: 15 minutes

18. Shrimp and Vegetable Stir-Fry

Ingredients:

- 1/2 lb shrimp, peeled and deveined
- 2 cups broccoli florets
- 1 bell pepper, thinly sliced
- 1 carrot, julienned
- 1/2 cup snap peas, trimmed
- 2 cloves garlic, minced
- 2 tablespoons low-sodium soy sauce
- 1 tablespoon hoisin sauce
- 1 tablespoon sesame oil

- 1 tablespoon green onions, sliced

- Sesame seeds for garnish

Instructions:

- In a wok or large skillet, heat sesame oil over medium-high heat.

- Add shrimp and stir-fry until pink and opaque, then set aside.

- In the same skillet, stir-fry broccoli, bell pepper, carrot, snap peas, and minced garlic until vegetables are crisp-tender.

- Add cooked shrimp back to the skillet.

- In a small bowl, mix soy sauce and hoisin sauce, then pour over the shrimp and vegetables.

- Toss everything together until well coated.

- Garnish with sliced green onions and sesame seeds before serving.

Nutritional Value:

- Calories: 320
- Protein: 20g
- Fiber: 7g
- Vitamin C: 80mg

Health Benefits:

- Shrimp provides lean protein.

- Vegetables offer a variety of vitamins and minerals.
- Sesame oil adds a touch of healthy fats.

Preparation Time: 20 minutes

19. Quinoa and Black Bean Stuffed Peppers

Ingredients:

- 4 bell peppers, halved and seeds removed
- 1 cup quinoa, cooked
- 1 can (15 oz) black beans, drained and rinsed
- 1 cup corn kernels (fresh or frozen)
- 1 cup diced tomatoes
- 1/2 cup red onion, finely chopped
- 1 teaspoon ground cumin
- 1/2 teaspoon chili powder
- Salt and pepper to taste
- Fresh cilantro for garnish

Instructions:

- Preheat the oven to 375°F (190°C).
- In a large bowl, combine cooked quinoa, black beans, corn, tomatoes, red onion, cumin, chili powder, salt, and pepper.
- Spoon the quinoa mixture into each bell pepper half.
- Place stuffed peppers in a baking dish.

- Cover with foil and bake for 25-30 minutes or until peppers are tender.
- Garnish with fresh cilantro before serving.

Nutritional Value:

- Calories: 320
- Protein: 14g
- Fiber: 9g
- Vitamin C: 120mg

Health Benefits:

- Quinoa provides a complete protein source.
- Bell peppers offer vitamin C and antioxidants.
- Black beans contribute fiber for digestive health.

Preparation Time: 40 minutes

20. Chicken and Vegetable Skewers

Ingredients:

- 1 lb boneless, skinless chicken breasts, cut into cubes
- 1 zucchini, sliced
- 1 bell pepper, cut into chunks
- 1 red onion, cut into wedges
- Cherry tomatoes
- 2 tablespoons olive oil

- 1 teaspoon dried oregano
- 1 teaspoon smoked paprika
- Salt and pepper to taste
- Lemon wedges for serving

Instructions:

- Preheat the grill or grill pan over medium-high heat.
- In a bowl, combine chicken cubes, zucchini slices, bell pepper chunks, red onion wedges, and cherry tomatoes.
- In a small bowl, mix olive oil, dried oregano, smoked paprika, salt, and pepper.
- Thread the chicken and vegetables onto skewers, alternating for variety.
- Brush the skewers with the olive oil mixture.
- Grill the skewers for 10-12 minutes, turning occasionally, until the chicken is cooked through.
- Serve with lemon wedges for a zesty touch.

Nutritional Value:

- Calories: 280
- Protein: 30g
- Healthy Fats: 10g
- Vitamin A: 600 IU

Health Benefits:

- Chicken provides lean protein.
- Vegetables offer essential vitamins and minerals.
- Olive oil contributes heart-healthy monounsaturated fats.

Preparation Time: 30 minutes

Dinner Creations

21. Baked Salmon with Lemon and Dill

Ingredients:

- 2 salmon fillets (6 oz each)
- 1 lemon, thinly sliced
- 2 tablespoons fresh dill, chopped
- 1 tablespoon olive oil
- 1 teaspoon garlic powder
- Salt and pepper to taste

Instructions:

- Preheat the oven to 400°F (200°C).
- Place the salmon fillets on a baking sheet lined with parchment paper.
- Drizzle olive oil over the salmon and season with garlic powder, salt, and pepper.

- Arrange lemon slices on top of each fillet and sprinkle with chopped dill.

- Bake for 15-20 minutes or until the salmon is cooked through and flakes easily.

- Serve with a side of steamed vegetables or quinoa.

Nutritional Value:

- Calories: 350
- Protein: 30g
- Omega-3 Fatty Acids: 1.5g
- Vitamin D: 10mcg

Health Benefits:

- Salmon provides omega-3 fatty acids for brain health.
- Dill adds a burst of flavor and has potential anti-inflammatory properties.

Preparation Time: 25 minutes

22. Mediterranean Chicken Bowl

Ingredients:

- 2 boneless, skinless chicken breasts
- 1 cup cherry tomatoes, halved
- 1 cucumber, diced
- 1/2 cup Kalamata olives, sliced

- 1/4 cup feta cheese, crumbled
- 2 tablespoons extra virgin olive oil
- 1 tablespoon balsamic vinegar
- 1 teaspoon dried oregano
- Salt and pepper to taste

Instructions:

- Season the chicken breasts with salt, pepper, and dried oregano.
- Grill or pan-sear the chicken until fully cooked, about 6-8 minutes per side.
- Slice the cooked chicken into strips.
- In a bowl, combine cherry tomatoes, cucumber, Kalamata olives, and feta cheese.
- Drizzle with olive oil and balsamic vinegar, tossing gently.
- Top the vegetable mixture with sliced grilled chicken.
- Serve as a Mediterranean-inspired chicken bowl.

Nutritional Value:

- Calories: 400
- Protein: 35g
- Fiber: 5g
- Healthy Fats: 18g

Health Benefits:

- Chicken provides lean protein.
- Mediterranean ingredients offer antioxidants and healthy fats.

Preparation Time: 30 minutes

23. Veggie and Quinoa Stuffed Bell Peppers

Ingredients:

- 4 bell peppers, halved and seeds removed
- 1 cup quinoa, cooked
- 1 can (15 oz) black beans, drained and rinsed
- 1 cup corn kernels (fresh or frozen)
- 1 cup diced tomatoes
- 1/2 cup red onion, finely chopped
- 1 teaspoon ground cumin
- 1/2 teaspoon chili powder
- Salt and pepper to taste
- Fresh cilantro for garnish

Instructions:

- Preheat the oven to 375°F (190°C).
- In a large bowl, combine cooked quinoa, black beans, corn, tomatoes, red onion, cumin, chili powder, salt, and pepper.

- Spoon the quinoa mixture into each bell pepper half.

- Place stuffed peppers in a baking dish.

- Cover with foil and bake for 25-30 minutes or until peppers are tender.

- Garnish with fresh cilantro before serving.

Nutritional Value:

- Calories: 320

- Protein: 14g

- Fiber: 9g

- Vitamin C: 120mg

Health Benefits:

- Quinoa provides a complete protein source.

- Bell peppers offer vitamin C and antioxidants.

- Black beans contribute fiber for digestive health.

Preparation Time: 40 minutes

24. Grilled Lemon Herb Chicken Skewers

Ingredients:

- 1 lb boneless, skinless chicken thighs, cut into cubes

- 1 zucchini, sliced

- 1 bell pepper, cut into chunks

- 1 red onion, cut into wedges

- Cherry tomatoes
- 2 tablespoons olive oil
- 1 lemon, juiced
- 1 teaspoon dried thyme
- 1 teaspoon dried rosemary
- Salt and pepper to taste
- Fresh parsley for garnish

Instructions:

- Preheat the grill or grill pan over medium-high heat.
- In a bowl, combine chicken cubes, zucchini slices, bell pepper chunks, red onion wedges, and cherry tomatoes.
- In a small bowl, whisk together olive oil, lemon juice, dried thyme, dried rosemary, salt, and pepper.
- Thread the chicken and vegetables onto skewers, alternating for variety.
- Brush the skewers with the olive oil mixture.
- Grill the skewers for 10-12 minutes, turning occasionally, until the chicken is cooked through.
- Garnish with fresh parsley before serving.

Nutritional Value:

- Calories: 300
- Protein: 25g

- Healthy Fats: 12g

- Vitamin C: 40mg

Health Benefits:

- Chicken provides lean protein.

- Vegetables offer essential vitamins and minerals.

- Lemon and herbs add refreshing flavors.

Preparation Time: 30 minutes

25. Quinoa and Chickpea Buddha Bowl

Ingredients:

- 1 cup cooked quinoa

- 1 can (15 oz) chickpeas, drained and rinsed

- 1 cup kale, chopped

- 1/2 cup shredded carrots

- 1/2 cucumber, sliced

- 1/4 cup hummus

- 2 tablespoons tahini

- 1 tablespoon lemon juice

- Salt and pepper to taste

- Sesame seeds for garnish

Instructions:

- In a bowl, arrange cooked quinoa, chickpeas, kale, shredded carrots, and cucumber.
- In a small bowl, whisk together hummus, tahini, lemon juice, salt, and pepper.
- Drizzle the dressing over the bowl.
- Garnish with sesame seeds for added crunch and flavor.
- Enjoy this nutrient-packed Buddha Bowl.

Nutritional Value:

- Calories: 380
- Protein: 15g
- Fiber: 12g
- Healthy Fats: 14g

Health Benefits:

- Quinoa provides a complete protein source.
- Chickpeas contribute plant-based protein and fiber.
- Kale offers a rich source of vitamins A and K.

Preparation Time: 20 minutes

26. Turkey and Vegetable Stir-Fry

Ingredients:

- 1 lb ground turkey
- 2 cups broccoli florets
- 1 bell pepper, thinly sliced
- 1 carrot, julienned
- 1/2 cup snap peas, trimmed
- 2 cloves garlic, minced
- 2 tablespoons low-sodium soy sauce
- 1 tablespoon hoisin sauce
- 1 tablespoon sesame oil
- 1 tablespoon green onions, sliced
- Sesame seeds for garnish

Instructions:

- In a large skillet, heat sesame oil over medium-high heat.
- Add ground turkey and cook until browned.
- Add broccoli, bell pepper, carrot, snap peas, and minced garlic to the skillet.
- Stir-fry until vegetables are crisp-tender.
- In a small bowl, mix soy sauce and hoisin sauce, then pour over the turkey and vegetables.
- Toss everything together until well coated.

- Garnish with sliced green onions and sesame seeds before serving.

Nutritional Value:

- Calories: 340
- Protein: 28g
- Fiber: 7g
- Vitamin C: 90mg

Health Benefits:

- Turkey provides lean protein.
- Vegetables offer essential vitamins and minerals.
- Sesame oil adds a touch of healthy fats.

Preparation Time: 25 minutes

27. Lentil and Vegetable Curry

Ingredients:

- 1 cup dry green lentils, rinsed
- 2 cups cauliflower florets
- 1 cup sweet potatoes, diced
- 1 can (14 oz) diced tomatoes, undrained
- 1 onion, finely chopped
- 3 cloves garlic, minced
- 1 tablespoon curry powder

- 1 teaspoon ground cumin
- 1 teaspoon ground turmeric
- 1/2 teaspoon cayenne pepper (adjust to taste)
- 1 can (14 oz) light coconut milk
- Salt and pepper to taste
- Fresh cilantro for garnish

Instructions:

- In a large pot, combine lentils, cauliflower, sweet potatoes, diced tomatoes, onion, garlic, curry powder, cumin, turmeric, and cayenne pepper.
- Pour in the light coconut milk and add salt and pepper to taste.
- Bring the mixture to a boil, then reduce the heat, cover, and simmer for 25-30 minutes or until lentils and vegetables are tender.
- Stir occasionally to prevent sticking.
- Garnish with fresh cilantro before serving.
- Serve over brown rice or quinoa.

Nutritional Value:

- Calories: 380
- Protein: 18g
- Fiber: 14g

- Vitamin A: 180% DV

Health Benefits:

- Lentils provide plant-based protein and fiber.
- Cauliflower and sweet potatoes offer vitamins and antioxidants.
- Turmeric has anti-inflammatory properties.

Preparation Time: 40 minutes

28. Lemon Herb Baked Cod

Ingredients:

- 4 cod fillets (6 oz each)
- 1 lemon, juiced and zested
- 2 tablespoons fresh parsley, chopped
- 1 tablespoon olive oil
- 2 cloves garlic, minced
- 1 teaspoon dried thyme
- Salt and pepper to taste
- Lemon wedges for serving

Instructions:

- Preheat the oven to 375°F (190°C).
- Place cod fillets on a baking sheet lined with parchment paper.

- In a small bowl, mix together lemon juice, lemon zest, parsley, olive oil, minced garlic, thyme, salt, and pepper.

- Brush the lemon herb mixture over each cod fillet.

- Bake for 15-20 minutes or until the cod is opaque and flakes easily.

- Serve with additional lemon wedges for a burst of citrus flavor.

Nutritional Value:

- Calories: 280
- Protein: 30g
- Healthy Fats: 10g
- Vitamin C: 30mg

Health Benefits:

- Cod provides lean protein and omega-3 fatty acids.
- Lemon and herbs add fresh and savory flavors.

Preparation Time: 25 minutes

29. Chickpea and Spinach Stuffed Acorn Squash

Ingredients:

- 2 acorn squash, halved and seeds removed
- 1 can (15 oz) chickpeas, drained and rinsed
- 2 cups fresh spinach, chopped

- 1/2 cup red onion, finely chopped
- 1/4 cup dried cranberries
- 1/4 cup walnuts, chopped
- 2 tablespoons olive oil
- 1 teaspoon ground cinnamon
- Salt and pepper to taste

Instructions:

- Preheat the oven to 400°F (200°C).
- Place acorn squash halves on a baking sheet.
- In a bowl, mix chickpeas, spinach, red onion, dried cranberries, walnuts, olive oil, cinnamon, salt, and pepper.
- Stuff each acorn squash half with the chickpea and spinach mixture.
- Bake for 30-40 minutes or until the squash is tender.
- Serve as a flavorful and nutritious dinner option.

Nutritional Value:

- Calories: 350
- Protein: 12g
- Fiber: 10g
- Vitamin A: 400% DV

Health Benefits:

- Chickpeas provide plant-based protein and fiber.

- Spinach offers vitamins A and K.

- Walnuts contribute omega-3 fatty acids.

Preparation Time: 45 minutes

30. Shrimp and Vegetable Stir-Fry

Ingredients:

- 1 lb shrimp, peeled and deveined

- 2 cups broccoli florets

- 1 bell pepper, thinly sliced

- 1 zucchini, sliced

- 2 carrots, julienned

- 3 cloves garlic, minced

- 2 tablespoons low-sodium soy sauce

- 1 tablespoon hoisin sauce

- 1 tablespoon sesame oil

- 1 tablespoon fresh ginger, grated

- Green onions for garnish

Instructions:

- In a wok or large skillet, heat sesame oil over medium-high heat.

- Add shrimp and stir-fry until pink and opaque. Remove from the wok and set aside.
- In the same wok, add broccoli, bell pepper, zucchini, carrots, garlic, and ginger. Stir-fry until vegetables are crisp-tender.
- In a small bowl, mix soy sauce and hoisin sauce, then add to the vegetable mixture.
- Return the cooked shrimp to the wok and toss everything until well coated.
- Garnish with green onions before serving.

Nutritional Value:

- Calories: 290
- Protein: 25g
- Fiber: 6g
- Vitamin C: 80mg

Health Benefits:

- Shrimp provides lean protein.
- Vegetables offer essential vitamins and minerals.
- Ginger adds a zesty flavor and potential anti-inflammatory properties.

Preparation Time: 20 minutes

31. Greek Yogurt Parfait

Ingredients:

- 1 cup low-fat Greek yogurt
- 1/2 cup mixed berries (blueberries, strawberries, raspberries)
- 1/4 cup granola (low-sugar)
- 1 tablespoon honey
- 1 tablespoon chopped nuts (almonds or walnuts)

Instructions:

- In a glass or bowl, layer the bottom with Greek yogurt.
- Add a layer of mixed berries on top of the yogurt.
- Sprinkle granola evenly over the berries.
- Drizzle honey over the granola layer.
- Top with chopped nuts for added crunch.
- Repeat the layers if desired.
- Serve immediately and enjoy this wholesome Greek Yogurt Parfait.

Nutritional Value:

- Calories: 250
- Protein: 15g
- Fiber: 4g

- Calcium: 200mg

Health Benefits:

- Greek yogurt provides protein and probiotics for gut health.
- Berries offer antioxidants and vitamins.
- Nuts contribute healthy fats and additional protein.

Preparation Time: 5 minutes

32. Avocado and Tomato Salsa

Ingredients:

- 1 ripe avocado, diced
- 1 cup cherry tomatoes, quartered
- 1/4 cup red onion, finely chopped
- 1/4 cup fresh cilantro, chopped
- 1 lime, juiced
- Salt and pepper to taste
- Whole-grain pita chips for serving

Instructions:

- In a bowl, gently combine diced avocado, cherry tomatoes, red onion, and cilantro.
- Drizzle lime juice over the mixture and toss gently.
- Season with salt and pepper according to taste.
- Allow the salsa to sit for a few minutes to enhance flavors.

- Serve with whole-grain pita chips for a delightful and nutritious snack.

Nutritional Value:

- Calories: 180
- Fiber: 6g
- Vitamin C: 20mg
- Healthy Fats: 14g

Health Benefits:

- Avocado provides heart-healthy monounsaturated fats.
- Tomatoes offer vitamins and antioxidants.
- Whole-grain pita chips contribute fiber.

Preparation Time: 10 minutes

33. Hummus and Vegetable Dip

Ingredients:

- 1 cup hummus (store-bought or homemade)
- 1 cup baby carrots
- 1 cucumber, sliced
- 1 bell pepper (any color), cut into strips
- 1 cup cherry tomatoes

Instructions:

- Place the hummus in a bowl or spread it on a serving plate.
- Arrange baby carrots, cucumber slices, bell pepper strips, and cherry tomatoes around the hummus.
- Use the vegetables to scoop up the hummus and enjoy a satisfying and nutritious dip.
- This snack provides a balance of protein, healthy fats, and fiber.

Nutritional Value:

- Calories: 250
- Protein: 8g
- Fiber: 10g
- Vitamin A: 170% DV

Health Benefits:

- Hummus offers plant-based protein and healthy fats.
- Vegetables provide essential vitamins and minerals.
- A well-rounded snack for brain health.

Preparation Time: 5 minutes

34. Apple and Almond Butter Sandwiches

Ingredients:

- 2 apples, cored and sliced horizontally into rounds
- 1/4 cup almond butter (unsweetened)
- 2 tablespoons chia seeds
- 2 tablespoons unsweetened shredded coconut

Instructions:

- Spread almond butter on half of the apple slices.
- Sprinkle chia seeds and shredded coconut evenly over the almond butter.
- Top with the remaining apple slices to create apple and almond butter sandwiches.
- Press gently to secure the sandwiches.
- This snack provides a combination of healthy fats, fiber, and protein.

Nutritional Value:

- Calories: 280
- Protein: 6g
- Fiber: 10g
- Healthy Fats: 15g

Health Benefits:

- Apples offer fiber and antioxidants.

- Almond butter provides protein and monounsaturated fats.

- Chia seeds contribute omega-3 fatty acids and additional fiber.

Preparation Time: 8 minutes

35. Cottage Cheese and Pineapple Bowls

Ingredients:

- 1 cup low-fat cottage cheese

- 1 cup fresh pineapple chunks

- 1/4 cup unsalted sunflower seeds

- 1 tablespoon honey (optional)

Instructions:

- In a bowl, combine cottage cheese and fresh pineapple chunks.

- Sprinkle sunflower seeds on top for added crunch and healthy fats.

- Drizzle honey over the mixture if you prefer a touch of sweetness.

- Gently toss the ingredients together.

- Serve in individual bowls for a satisfying and protein-rich snack.

Nutritional Value:

- Calories: 280
- Protein: 18g
- Fiber: 3g
- Vitamin C: 50mg

Health Benefits:

- Cottage cheese provides a good source of protein and calcium.
- Pineapple offers vitamin C and digestive enzymes.
- Sunflower seeds contribute healthy fats and additional protein.

Preparation Time: 5 minutes

36. Guacamole and Whole Grain Pita

Ingredients:

- 2 ripe avocados, mashed
- 1 tomato, diced
- 1/4 cup red onion, finely chopped
- 1 clove garlic, minced
- 1 lime, juiced

- Salt and pepper to taste
- Whole grain pita bread, cut into triangles

Instructions:

- In a bowl, combine mashed avocados, diced tomato, red onion, minced garlic, lime juice, salt, and pepper.
- Mix the ingredients until well combined.
- Serve the guacamole with whole grain pita triangles.
- This snack provides healthy fats, fiber, and essential nutrients.

Nutritional Value:

- Calories: 220
- Fiber: 8g
- Healthy Fats: 15g
- Vitamin K: 30% DV

Health Benefits:

- Avocados offer monounsaturated fats and potassium.
- Tomatoes provide antioxidants and vitamins.
- Whole grain pita adds fiber for sustained energy.

Preparation Time: 10 minutes

37. Cucumber and Salmon Bites

Ingredients:

- 1 cucumber, sliced into rounds
- 4 oz smoked salmon, cut into small pieces
- 2 tablespoons Greek yogurt
- 1 teaspoon capers
- Fresh dill for garnish

Instructions:

- Place cucumber rounds on a serving platter.
- Top each cucumber round with a small piece of smoked salmon.
- Add a small dollop of Greek yogurt on top of the salmon.
- Garnish with capers and fresh dill.
- These bite-sized snacks offer a combination of omega-3 fatty acids, protein, and refreshing flavors.

Nutritional Value:

- Calories: 120
- Protein: 15g
- Healthy Fats: 4g
- Omega-3 Fatty Acids: 800mg

Health Benefits:

- Salmon provides omega-3 fatty acids for brain health.
- Greek yogurt offers protein and probiotics.
- Cucumbers add hydration and vitamins.

Preparation Time: 10 minutes

38. Berry and Almond Rice Cakes

Ingredients:

- 4 rice cakes (whole grain)
- 1/2 cup almond butter (unsweetened)
- 1 cup mixed berries (strawberries, blueberries, raspberries)
- 2 tablespoons chia seeds

Instructions:

- Spread almond butter evenly on each rice cake.
- Top the almond butter with mixed berries.
- Sprinkle chia seeds over the berries for added nutrition.
- These rice cake snacks provide a mix of healthy fats, fiber, and antioxidants.

Nutritional Value:

- Calories: 280
- Protein: 8g

- Fiber: 6g

- Healthy Fats: 16g

Health Benefits:

- Almond butter offers protein and monounsaturated fats.

- Berries provide antioxidants and vitamins.

- Chia seeds contribute omega-3 fatty acids and additional fiber.

Preparation Time: 8 minutes

39. Quinoa and Vegetable Stuffed Bell Peppers

Ingredients:

- 2 bell peppers, halved and seeds removed

- 1 cup cooked quinoa

- 1/2 cup black beans, drained and rinsed

- 1/2 cup corn kernels

- 1/4 cup red onion, finely chopped

- 1/4 cup fresh cilantro, chopped

- 1 lime, juiced

- 1 teaspoon cumin

- Salt and pepper to taste

Instructions:

- Preheat the oven to 375°F (190°C).

- In a bowl, mix cooked quinoa, black beans, corn, red onion, cilantro, lime juice, cumin, salt, and pepper.
- Stuff each bell pepper half with the quinoa and vegetable mixture.
- Place the stuffed peppers on a baking sheet.
- Bake for 20-25 minutes or until the peppers are tender.
- These stuffed bell peppers offer a balance of fiber, protein, and essential nutrients.

Nutritional Value:

- Calories: 280
- Protein: 12g
- Fiber: 8g
- Vitamin C: 120% DV

Health Benefits:

- Quinoa provides complete protein and fiber.
- Black beans offer additional protein and fiber.
- Bell peppers contribute vitamins A and C.

Preparation Time: 30 minutes

40. Mango Salsa with Whole Grain Tortilla Chips

Ingredients:

- 1 ripe mango, diced

- 1/2 cup red bell pepper, finely chopped

- 1/4 cup red onion, minced

- 1/4 cup fresh cilantro, chopped

- 1 jalapeño, seeds removed and minced

- 1 lime, juiced

- Whole grain tortilla chips for serving

Instructions:

- In a bowl, combine diced mango, red bell pepper, red onion, cilantro, jalapeño, and lime juice.

- Mix the ingredients until well combined.

- Allow the mango salsa to chill in the refrigerator for at least 15 minutes.

- Serve with whole grain tortilla chips for a refreshing and tangy snack.

- This snack provides vitamins, antioxidants, and a burst of tropical flavor.

Nutritional Value:

- Calories: 220

- Fiber: 5g

- Vitamin C: 60mg

Health Benefits:

- Mango offers vitamin A and antioxidants.
- Bell peppers contribute vitamin C.
- Whole grain tortilla chips provide fiber.

Preparation Time: 15 minutes

Delectable Dessert

41. Dark Chocolate-Dipped Strawberries

Ingredients:

- 1 cup fresh strawberries, washed and dried
- 3 oz dark chocolate (70% cocoa or higher)
- 1 tablespoon unsweetened shredded coconut (optional)
- 1 tablespoon chopped nuts (almonds or walnuts)

Instructions:

- Melt the dark chocolate in a heatproof bowl over simmering water or in the microwave using short intervals.
- Dip each strawberry into the melted chocolate, coating about two-thirds of the berry.
- Place the dipped strawberries on a parchment-lined tray.
- Sprinkle unsweetened shredded coconut or chopped nuts on top of the chocolate coating.

- Allow the chocolate to set in the refrigerator for at least 30 minutes.
- These dark chocolate-dipped strawberries offer antioxidants, vitamins, and a touch of sweetness.

Nutritional Value:

- Calories: 150
- Fiber: 4g
- Vitamin C: 50mg
- Antioxidants: Flavonoids

Health Benefits:

- Dark chocolate provides flavonoids for heart health.
- Strawberries offer vitamin C and antioxidants.
- Nuts contribute healthy fats and additional nutrients.

Preparation Time: 15 minutes

42. Greek Yogurt and Berry Parfait

Ingredients:

- 1 cup low-fat Greek yogurt
- 1/2 cup mixed berries (blueberries, raspberries, blackberries)
- 1 tablespoon honey (optional)
- 2 tablespoons granola (low-sugar)
- Fresh mint leaves for garnish

Instructions:

- In a glass or bowl, layer the bottom with low-fat Greek yogurt.
- Add a layer of mixed berries on top of the yogurt.
- Drizzle honey over the berries if additional sweetness is desired.
- Sprinkle granola evenly over the berries.
- Repeat the layers if desired.
- Garnish with fresh mint leaves for a refreshing touch.
- Serve immediately, providing probiotics, antioxidants, and fiber.

Nutritional Value:

- Calories: 220
- Protein: 15g
- Fiber: 3g
- Probiotics: Lactic Acid Bacteria

Health Benefits:

- Greek yogurt offers probiotics for gut health.
- Berries provide antioxidants and vitamins.
- Granola adds fiber and crunch.

Preparation Time: 10 minutes

43. Banana and Almond Butter Bites

Ingredients:

- 2 bananas, peeled and sliced into rounds
- 2 tablespoons almond butter (unsweetened)
- 2 tablespoons unsweetened shredded coconut
- 2 tablespoons chopped almonds

Instructions:

- Spread almond butter on one side of each banana round.
- Press two almond-butter-coated banana rounds together to form a bite-sized sandwich.
- Roll the edges of the banana bites in shredded coconut and chopped almonds.
- Place the prepared bites on a tray lined with parchment paper.
- Chill in the refrigerator for at least 30 minutes before serving.
- These banana and almond butter bites offer a combination of healthy fats, potassium, and a natural sweetness.

Nutritional Value:

- Calories: 180
- Protein: 5g
- Healthy Fats: 8g

- Potassium: 450mg

Health Benefits:

- Bananas provide potassium and natural sugars.

- Almond butter offers protein and monounsaturated fats.

- Shredded coconut and almonds add texture and additional nutrients.

Preparation Time: 15 minutes

44. Chia Seed Pudding with Mixed Berries

Ingredients:

- 1/4 cup chia seeds

- 1 cup unsweetened almond milk

- 1 tablespoon maple syrup (optional)

- 1/2 teaspoon vanilla extract

- 1/2 cup mixed berries (strawberries, blueberries, raspberries)

- Fresh mint leaves for garnish

Instructions:

- In a bowl, combine chia seeds, almond milk, maple syrup (if using), and vanilla extract.

- Stir well and let the mixture sit for 10 minutes, stirring occasionally.

- Cover the bowl and refrigerate for at least 2 hours or overnight until the chia seeds absorb the liquid and create a pudding-like consistency.
- Before serving, layer the chia seed pudding with mixed berries.
- Garnish with fresh mint leaves for a burst of flavor.
- This chia seed pudding offers omega-3 fatty acids, fiber, and antioxidants.

Nutritional Value:

- Calories: 200
- Fiber: 10g
- Omega-3 Fatty Acids: 1,500mg

Health Benefits:

- Chia seeds provide omega-3 fatty acids and fiber.
- Almond milk offers a dairy-free alternative with added vitamins.
- Berries contribute antioxidants and vitamins.

Preparation Time: 15 minutes (excluding chilling time)

45. Baked Cinnamon Apples

Ingredients:

- 2 apples, cored and sliced

- 1 tablespoon melted coconut oil
- 1 teaspoon ground cinnamon
- 1 tablespoon chopped walnuts
- 1 tablespoon raisins

Instructions:

- Preheat the oven to 350°F (175°C).
- In a bowl, toss apple slices with melted coconut oil and ground cinnamon until evenly coated.
- Arrange the apple slices in a baking dish.
- Sprinkle chopped walnuts and raisins over the apples.
- Bake for 20-25 minutes or until the apples are tender.
- These baked cinnamon apples offer a warm and comforting dessert with added fiber and healthy fats.

Nutritional Value:

- Calories: 180
- Fiber: 6g
- Healthy Fats: 8g
- Vitamin C: 8mg

Health Benefits:

- Apples provide fiber and antioxidants.
- Walnuts offer omega-3 fatty acids and additional nutrients.

- Cinnamon adds flavor and potential anti-inflammatory properties.

Preparation Time: 25 minutes

46. Mango and Coconut Chia Popsicles

Ingredients:

- 1 cup diced mango
- 1/2 cup unsweetened coconut milk
- 2 tablespoons chia seeds
- 1 tablespoon honey (optional)

Instructions:

- In a blender, combine diced mango, coconut milk, chia seeds, and honey (if using).
- Blend until smooth.
- Pour the mixture into popsicle molds.
- Freeze for at least 4 hours or until solid.
- Run warm water over the molds to release the popsicles.
- These mango and coconut chia popsicles offer a refreshing and tropical treat with added fiber.

Nutritional Value:

- Calories: 120
- Fiber: 4g

- Vitamin A: 500 IU

Health Benefits:

- Mango provides vitamin A and antioxidants.
- Chia seeds offer omega-3 fatty acids and fiber.
- Coconut milk adds a creamy texture with healthy fats.

Preparation Time: 10 minutes (excluding freezing time)

47. Berry and Oatmeal Crumble

Ingredients:

- 1 cup mixed berries (blueberries, raspberries, blackberries)
- 1 tablespoon maple syrup
- 1 tablespoon whole wheat flour
- 1/2 cup old-fashioned oats
- 2 tablespoons chopped almonds
- 1 tablespoon coconut oil, melted

Instructions:

- Preheat the oven to 375°F (190°C).
- In a bowl, mix mixed berries with maple syrup and whole wheat flour.
- In a separate bowl, combine oats, chopped almonds, and melted coconut oil.

- Spread the berry mixture in a baking dish and sprinkle the oat topping evenly.

- Bake for 20-25 minutes or until the top is golden brown.

- Allow it to cool slightly before serving.

- This berry and oatmeal crumble provide antioxidants, fiber, and healthy fats.

Nutritional Value:

- Calories: 200

- Fiber: 8g

- Healthy Fats: 9g

- Antioxidants: Anthocyanins

Health Benefits:

- Berries offer antioxidants and vitamins.

- Oats provide fiber and sustained energy.

- Almonds contribute healthy fats and additional nutrients.

Preparation Time: 30 minutes

48. Avocado Chocolate Mousse

Ingredients:

- 2 ripe avocados, peeled and pitted

- 1/4 cup unsweetened cocoa powder

- 1/4 cup honey or maple syrup

- 1 teaspoon vanilla extract
- Pinch of sea salt
- Fresh berries for garnish

Instructions:

- In a blender or food processor, combine avocados, cocoa powder, honey or maple syrup, vanilla extract, and a pinch of sea salt.
- Blend until smooth and creamy.
- Divide the mousse into serving bowls.
- Refrigerate for at least 1-hour before serving.
- Garnish with fresh berries before serving.
- This avocado chocolate mousse offers a rich and indulgent treat with heart-healthy fats.

Nutritional Value:

- Calories: 180
- Fiber: 7g
- Healthy Fats: 14g
- Vitamin E: 4mg

Health Benefits:

- Avocados provide monounsaturated fats and vitamin E.

- Cocoa powder offers antioxidants and potential mood-boosting compounds.
- Honey or maple syrup adds natural sweetness.

Preparation Time: 15 minutes

49. Almond and Apricot Energy Bites

Ingredients:

- 1 cup dried apricots, unsweetened
- 1 cup almonds
- 1/4 cup chia seeds
- 1 teaspoon almond extract
- 1/4 cup shredded coconut (unsweetened)
- A pinch of sea salt

Instructions:

- In a food processor, combine dried apricots, almonds, chia seeds, almond extract, and a pinch of sea salt.
- Blend until the mixture forms a sticky dough.
- Roll the dough into bite-sized balls.
- Roll each energy bite in shredded coconut to coat.
- Place the bites on a tray and refrigerate for at least 30 minutes.
- These almond and apricot energy bites offer a delightful blend of natural sweetness and healthy fats.

Nutritional Value:

- Calories: 150

- Protein: 4g

- Healthy Fats: 9g

- Fiber: 5g

Health Benefits:

- Apricots provide fiber, potassium, and vitamins.

- Almonds offer protein, monounsaturated fats, and vitamin E.

- Chia seeds contribute omega-3 fatty acids and additional fiber.

Preparation Time: 20 minutes

50. Coconut Yogurt Parfait

Ingredients:

- 1 cup coconut yogurt (unsweetened)

- 1/2 cup pineapple chunks

- 2 tablespoons shredded coconut (unsweetened)

- 1 tablespoon chopped macadamia nuts

- 1 teaspoon honey (optional)

Instructions:

- In a glass or bowl, layer coconut yogurt, pineapple chunks, and shredded coconut.
- Repeat the layers if desired.
- Top the parfait with chopped macadamia nuts.
- Drizzle honey over the parfait for added sweetness if desired.
- Serve immediately for a tropical and satisfying dessert.

Nutritional Value:

- Calories: 200
- Fiber: 6g
- Healthy Fats: 12g

Health Benefits:

- Coconut yogurt provides probiotics and healthy fats.
- Pineapple offers vitamins, enzymes, and antioxidants.
- Macadamia nuts contribute monounsaturated fats and additional nutrients.

Preparation Time: 10 minutes

51. Berry Bliss Smoothie

Ingredients:

- 1/2 cup mixed berries (blueberries, strawberries, raspberries)
- 1/2 banana, frozen
- 1/2 cup low-fat Greek yogurt
- 1 tablespoon chia seeds
- 1/2 cup unsweetened almond milk
- Ice cubes (optional)

Instructions:

- In a blender, combine mixed berries, frozen banana, Greek yogurt, chia seeds, and almond milk.
- Blend until smooth and creamy.
- Add ice cubes if a colder consistency is desired.
- Pour into a glass and serve immediately.
- This Berry Bliss Smoothie provides antioxidants, probiotics, and omega-3 fatty acids.

Nutritional Value:

- Calories: 180
- Protein: 10g
- Fiber: 6g

- Omega-3 Fatty Acids: 1,000mg

Health Benefits:

- Mixed berries offer antioxidants and vitamins.

- Greek yogurt provides probiotics and protein.

- Chia seeds contribute omega-3 fatty acids and additional fiber.

Preparation Time: 5 minutes

52. Green Citrus Burst Juice

Ingredients:

- 1 cup kale leaves, stems removed

- 1/2 cucumber, peeled and sliced

- 1 green apple, cored and sliced

- 1/2 lemon, peeled

- 1-inch piece of ginger, peeled

- 1 cup water or coconut water

- Ice cubes (optional)

Instructions:

- In a juicer, process kale, cucumber, green apple, lemon, and ginger.

- Collect the juice in a glass.

- Dilute with water or coconut water according to taste preference.

- Add ice cubes if desired for a chilled beverage.

- This Green Citrus Burst Juice offers vitamins, minerals, and hydration.

Nutritional Value:

- Calories: 80
- Vitamin C: 60mg
- Vitamin K: 120mcg
- Hydration: 1 cup

Health Benefits:

- Kale provides vitamin K and antioxidants.
- Cucumber offers hydration and additional vitamins.
- Lemon and ginger add flavor and potential anti-inflammatory properties.

Preparation Time: 7 minutes

53. Tropical Turmeric Smoothie

Ingredients:

- 1/2 cup pineapple chunks
- 1/2 cup mango chunks
- 1/2 banana, frozen

- 1/2 teaspoon turmeric powder
- 1/2 teaspoon ginger, grated
- 1 cup coconut water
- Ice cubes (optional)

Instructions:

- In a blender, combine pineapple chunks, mango chunks, frozen banana, turmeric powder, grated ginger, and coconut water.
- Blend until smooth.
- Add ice cubes if a colder consistency is desired.
- Pour into a glass and serve immediately.
- This Tropical Turmeric Smoothie provides anti-inflammatory benefits, vitamins, and hydration.

Nutritional Value:

- Calories: 150
- Vitamin C: 40mg
- Potassium: 400mg
- Anti-Inflammatory Compounds: Curcumin

Health Benefits:

- Pineapple and mango offer vitamins and antioxidants.

- Turmeric provides curcumin with potential anti-inflammatory properties.

- Coconut water adds hydration and electrolytes.

Preparation Time: 6 minutes

54. Berry Avocado Delight Smoothie

Ingredients:

- 1/2 cup mixed berries (blueberries, raspberries, strawberries)

- 1/2 avocado, peeled and pitted

- 1/2 cup spinach leaves

- 1/2 cup almond milk (unsweetened)

- 1 tablespoon flaxseeds

- Ice cubes (optional)

Instructions:

- In a blender, combine mixed berries, avocado, spinach leaves, almond milk, and flaxseeds.

- Blend until smooth.

- Add ice cubes if a colder consistency is desired.

- Pour into a glass and serve immediately.

- This Berry Avocado Delight Smoothie provides healthy fats, antioxidants, and fiber.

Nutritional Value:

- Calories: 200
- Fiber: 7g
- Healthy Fats: 12g
- Vitamins: A, C, K

Health Benefits:

- Mixed berries offer antioxidants and vitamins.
- Avocado provides monounsaturated fats and additional nutrients.
- Flaxseeds contribute omega-3 fatty acids and fiber.

Preparation Time: 7 minutes

55. Citrus Mint Refresh Smoothie

Ingredients:

- 1/2 cup orange segments
- 1/2 cup cucumber, peeled and sliced
- 1/2 cup fresh mint leaves
- 1/2 banana, frozen
- 1/2 cup plain Greek yogurt
- 1/2 cup water
- Ice cubes (optional)

Instructions:

- In a blender, combine orange segments, cucumber, mint leaves, frozen banana, Greek yogurt, and water.
- Blend until smooth.
- Add ice cubes if a colder consistency is desired.
- Pour into a glass and serve immediately.
- This Citrus Mint Refresh Smoothie provides vitamin C, hydration, and probiotics.

Nutritional Value:

- Calories: 120
- Vitamin C: 45mg
- Probiotics: 5g
- Hydration: 1/2 cup

Health Benefits:

- Oranges offer vitamin C and antioxidants.
- Cucumber provides hydration and additional vitamins.
- Greek yogurt adds probiotics and protein.

Preparation Time: 5 minutes

56. Peach Almond Bliss Smoothie

Ingredients:

- 1/2 cup sliced peaches (fresh or frozen)
- 1/2 cup almond milk (unsweetened)
- 1/2 cup baby spinach leaves
- 1/4 cup almonds
- 1 tablespoon honey (optional)
- 1/2 teaspoon vanilla extract
- Ice cubes (optional)

Instructions:

- In a blender, combine sliced peaches, almond milk, baby spinach leaves, almonds, honey (if using), and vanilla extract.
- Blend until smooth.
- Add ice cubes if a colder consistency is desired.
- Pour into a glass and serve immediately.
- This Peach Almond Bliss Smoothie provides vitamins, minerals, and healthy fats.

Nutritional Value:

- Calories: 180
- Vitamin A: 2,000 IU

- Healthy Fats: 8g

- Fiber: 4g

Health Benefits:

- Peaches offer vitamins and antioxidants.

- Almond milk provides a dairy-free source of calcium.

- Spinach adds additional vitamins and minerals.

Preparation Time: 6 minutes

57. Blueberry Basil Bliss Smoothie

Ingredients:

- 1/2 cup blueberries (fresh or frozen)

- 1/2 cup strawberries, hulled

- 1/2 cup fresh basil leaves

- 1/2 banana, frozen

- 1/2 cup coconut water

- 1 tablespoon chia seeds

- Ice cubes (optional)

Instructions:

- In a blender, combine blueberries, strawberries, fresh basil leaves, frozen banana, coconut water, and chia seeds.

- Blend until smooth.

- Add ice cubes if a colder consistency is desired.

- Pour into a glass and serve immediately.
- This Blueberry Basil Bliss Smoothie provides antioxidants, hydration, and omega-3 fatty acids.

Nutritional Value:

- Calories: 150
- Antioxidants: Anthocyanins
- Omega-3 Fatty Acids: 1,000mg
- Hydration: 1/2 cup

Health Benefits:

- Blueberries offer antioxidants and vitamins.
- Basil provides additional antioxidants and potential anti-inflammatory properties.
- Chia seeds contribute omega-3 fatty acids and fiber.

Preparation Time: 5 minutes

58. Pineapple Coconut Elixir Smoothie

Ingredients:

- 1/2 cup pineapple chunks
- 1/2 cup coconut milk (unsweetened)
- 1/2 cup kale leaves, stems removed
- 1/2 avocado, peeled and pitted
- 1 tablespoon hemp seeds

- 1 teaspoon lime juice

- Ice cubes (optional)

Instructions:

- In a blender, combine pineapple chunks, coconut milk, kale leaves, avocado, hemp seeds, and lime juice.

- Blend until smooth.

- Add ice cubes if a colder consistency is desired.

- Pour into a glass and serve immediately.

- This Pineapple Coconut Elixir Smoothie provides vitamins, healthy fats, and omega-3 fatty acids.

Nutritional Value:

- Calories: 180

- Vitamin C: 45mg

- Healthy Fats: 10g

- Omega-3 Fatty Acids: 1,500mg

Health Benefits:

- Pineapple offers vitamin C and digestive enzymes.

- Coconut milk provides healthy fats.

- Kale adds vitamins, minerals, and fiber.

Preparation Time: 6 minutes

59. Mango Turmeric Tango Smoothie

Ingredients:

- 1/2 cup mango chunks
- 1/2 cup pineapple chunks
- 1/2 teaspoon turmeric powder
- 1/2 teaspoon ginger, grated
- 1/2 cup almond milk (unsweetened)
- 1 tablespoon flaxseeds
- Ice cubes (optional)

Instructions:

- In a blender, combine mango chunks, pineapple chunks, turmeric powder, grated ginger, almond milk, and flaxseeds.
- Blend until smooth.
- Add ice cubes if a colder consistency is desired.
- Pour into a glass and serve immediately.
- This Mango Turmeric Tango Smoothie provides antioxidants, vitamins, and omega-3 fatty acids.

Nutritional Value:

- Calories: 160
- Antioxidants: Beta-carotene
- Omega-3 Fatty Acids: 1,200mg

- Fiber: 4g

Health Benefits:

- Mango and pineapple offer antioxidants and vitamins.
- Turmeric provides curcumin with potential anti-inflammatory properties.
- Flaxseeds contribute omega-3 fatty acids and fiber.

Preparation Time: 5 minutes

60. Raspberry Almond Joy Smoothie

Ingredients:

- 1/2 cup raspberries (fresh or frozen)
- 1/2 banana, frozen
- 1/2 cup almond butter
- 1 cup almond milk (unsweetened)
- 1 tablespoon cocoa powder (unsweetened)
- 1 tablespoon coconut flakes
- Ice cubes (optional)

Instructions:

In a blender, combine raspberries, frozen banana, almond butter, almond milk, cocoa powder, and coconut flakes.

Blend until smooth.

- Add ice cubes if a colder consistency is desired.

- Pour into a glass and serve immediately.

- This Raspberry Almond Joy Smoothie provides antioxidants, healthy fats, and a touch of sweetness.

Nutritional Value:

- Calories: 220

- Antioxidants: Polyphenols

- Healthy Fats: 14g

- Fiber: 5g

Health Benefits:

- Raspberries offer antioxidants and vitamins.

- Almond butter provides healthy fats and protein.

- Cocoa powder adds a rich flavor and potential mood-boosting benefits.

Preparation Time: 6 minutes

CONCLUSION

In concluding our journey through the "Complete Dash Diet Cookbook for Alzheimer's," we stand at the intersection of culinary delight and cognitive well-being. This cookbook transcends the realms of mere recipes; it becomes a compass guiding you towards a flavorful, brain-boosting lifestyle.

Our exploration into Dash diet-inspired meals for Alzheimer's has illuminated the potent connection between nutrition and cognitive health. Through carefully crafted recipes, we've harnessed the power of ingredients renowned for their brain-boosting properties, aligning seamlessly with the principles of the Dash diet.

As you embark on this culinary expedition, remember that each recipe is a step towards nurturing your cognitive vitality. Embrace the variety of flavors, textures, and nutrients presented in these pages. Let the colors on your plate symbolizes not only a feast for the senses but also a feast for your brain.

In the realm of Alzheimer's prevention, adopting a Dash diet is a proactive and pleasurable choice. The amalgamation of nutrient-dense foods, beneficial fats, and mindful preparation methods provides a blueprint for creating meals that contribute not only to your physical health but also to the resilience of your cognitive faculties.

May this cookbook serve as a trusted companion on your journey towards a brain-healthy lifestyle. As you savor the delectable offerings within these pages, envision each bite as a gesture of self-care and cognitive fortification. The kitchen transforms into a sanctuary where you craft not just meals but a defense against cognitive decline.

Embrace the joy of cooking, the nourishment of mindful eating, and the empowerment that comes with taking charge of your well-being. The "Complete Dash Diet Cookbook for Alzheimer's" is more than a collection of recipes; it's a celebration of the remarkable connection between the food we consume and the resilience of our minds.

Here's to savoring not just the flavors but the promise of cognitive wellness with every delectable dish.

Bon Appétit and Brain Health!